How To Choose Olive Oil

12 Impressive Health Benefits, And Some Precautions Of Olive Oil

By

Dr. Rebecca T. Luna

INTRODUCTION

The most frequently suggested oil by health advocates is olive oil. There are so many advantages to olive oil that it is not surprising that it

was referred to as liquid gold in ancient times. Your skin can benefit from this amazing oil.
It goes beyond just a simple kitchen essential.
Olive oil may help with weight loss, lower the risk of cancer and arthritis, and control cholesterol levels. Additionally, it controls blood sugar levels. Since it is mostly grown there, Mediterranean people drink the most olive oil. There are much fewer deaths from cardiovascular problems there than in other parts of the world, which demonstrates the beneficial effects of olive oil on health.
Are you prepared to discover the many advantages that this oil has to offer? Please scroll down to learn more about the advantages, applications, and dangers of olive oil.

CHAPTER 1

A quick Summary Of Olive Oil

Family: Oleaceae Scientific
Name: Olea europaea
Origin: Mediterranean Basin

The olive fruit is used to make olive oil. Olive oil has recently been popular all across the world, dominating everything from our kitchens to the world of cosmetics.

When you go shopping, you notice a wide selection of olive oils. The information you receive in the following few minutes will help you understand what they are all about.

Virgin Olive Oil: The most widely used type of olive oil, virgin olive oil has a remarkably low acid concentration for cooking oil. It is most appropriate for those who want to profit from olive oil without spending a fortune.

Extra Virgin Olive Oi: Is thought to be the greatest for our bodies because it is produced by cold pressing olive fruit. But keep in mind that because extra virgin oil is so expensive, not everyone can afford to use it.

Pure Olive Oil : This oil is a mixture of virgin and refined olive oils. Because of its high acid content, it cannot be used.

Lampante Oil: The kind of oil that is only used as fuel and not for cooking.
Let's move on to the advantages now that you are aware of the types.

The Numerous Advantages Of Olive Oil

Olive Oil Benefits The Skin

You're viewing a video on YouTube when an advertisement with a famous person gushing about her preferred skin cream and persuading you of its efficacy appears. You hurried to a cosmetic store to get the cream, only to discover that it is astronomically expensive. What if we told you that olive oil has many of the same advantages as some of the priciest cosmetic products available?

Here are some reasons why olive oil is better than all the skin lotions on the market that are full of chemicals.

Tip: Hydrates Skin
I want to ask you a few questions before we move on.
Do you always moisturize yourself at home after taking a shower?
Do you use up a bottle of lotion for your body within a month?

Are you open to using a natural lotion in place of your usual name-brand product? A treatment that has fewer side effects and will last longer? Choose olive oil if all or some of your answers to my questions were "yes."

Olive oil's high vitamin E concentration, an antioxidant that shields the skin from environmental aggressors like wind and sun, gives it nutritional benefits. Olive oil's non-sticky, light texture makes it ideal for all skin types as a long-lasting moisturizer that doesn't stick to the skin.

What You Require

1 teaspoon, Extra virgin olive oil

What You Should Do

• After taking a shower, massage some olive oil over your face while your skin is still slightly damp.

• After about 15 minutes, remove it by rinsing it with warm water.

Apply the oil to your face before bed and leave it on the night if you have dry skin. Using a mild face cleanser and some warm water, you may remove the oil in the morning.

CHAPTER 2

Tip: Enhances Skin Health

The majority of us swear by natural elements when it comes to beauty. All we desire is beautiful skin.

No matter how many creams you have on hand, we always turn to fruit pulp or vegetable juice extract for a quick treatment.

How does olive oil assist?

Vitamin E, which is present in olive oil, enhances skin health by reducing inflammation and acne and shielding the skin against dangerous conditions like psoriasis and skin cancer.
Yogurt works as a light exfoliator and honey as a humectant, improving the health of the skin.

What You Require

yogurt, 1/4 cup of honey, and 2 teaspoons of extra virgin olive oil

What You Should Do

Up until you get a thick solution, thoroughly combine the ingredients.

Apply this remedy to your face, then leave it on there for around 20 minutes.

With warm water, remove it.

This treatment can be used once each week.

Tip: Aids In n MakeUp Removal

Are you having trouble deciding which makeup remover to buy? Do not worry.

Virgin olive oil is a simple and inexpensive substitute for store brands. In addition, where can you get a solution that works without endangering your skin? Since I have sensitive skin that breaks out in rashes or blisters at the slightest difference in the goods, I always advise using natural solutions.

What You Require

13 cup yogurt, 14 cup honey, and 2 teaspoons of extra virgin olive oil

What You Should Do

To remove makeup, dip a few cotton balls in olive oil and rub your face with them.

You may also use a cotton pad dampened with olive oil to wipe away eye makeup. The oil can soften the skin around your eyes in addition to removing makeup.

Tip: Possesses Anti-Aging Qualities
Your skin begins to droop and wrinkle as you get older. Olive oil can help you postpone these aging symptoms.

What You Require
Olive oil, 2 tablespoons
Lemon juice, 1 tablespoon
a dash of salt, the sea

What You Should Do
Apply a few drops of olive oil to your face and massage it.
To make an exfoliant, combine the leftover oil and sea salt.
Add lemon juice to feel more refreshed.

Apply this combination to your face's dry, scaly, and rough spots.

CHAPTER 3

Tip: Maintains Hair Health

Olive oil may do wonders for your hair when combined with a few additional things. Vitamin E found in abundance in the oil helps prevent hair loss. Your hair is moisturized by honey. Additionally, it contains vitamins B, magnesium, zinc, sulfur, calcium, and other minerals that promote hair development. The main component of hair is protein, which is abundant in egg yolks.

What You Tequire
Olive oil, 1/2 cup
Honey, 2 tablespoons
egg yolk

What You Should Do

•Thoroughly combine the ingredients until you get a smooth paste.

• Apply this paste to your hair, then leave it in place for 20 minutes.

•Rinse with warm water, then use a conditioner afterward.

Your hair is moisturized by olive oil, which also soothes your itchy scalp.

Benefits Of Olive Oil For Health

Olive oil has many advantages besides just improving your appearance. A lot of health advantages can be obtained from consuming this oil in your diet as well.

Tip: Promotes Healthy Nails

Your nails are a great indicator of your health. Often, doctors will examine your nails if you appear pale. Nails that are lifeless, brittle, and dull are a few issues we run into. Olive oil, though, can enhance the health of your nails. You need to start taking care of your nails so they look healthy if you

want to sport that trendy nail art at your best friend's wedding.
The appearance of nails with a condition can be improved by vitamin E in olive oil

What hat You Require
Olive oil, two to three tablespoons

What You Should Do
1. Simply dab your nails with a cotton ball that has been dipped in olive oil.
2. Before washing it off with regular water, you can leave it on for about 30 minutes.

Tip: Aids in Breast Cancer Prevention
Oncology and olive oil The correlation could be described as ridiculous. However, using olive oil when you cook can help prevent breast cancer. Oleuropein, a naturally occurring substance found in olive leaves, was discovered to have potential anti-breast cancer properties in a Saudi Arabian study.

Another clinical trial carried out in Spain discovered that women who consumed olive oil in their diet had a 62 percent lower risk of developing breast cancer.

CHAPTER 4

Tip: Helps Prevent Diabetes

Incorporating olive oil into your diet is one of the best ways to maintain healthy blood sugar levels. Have faith in the numerous studies that have proven this one reality.

Olive oil is one of the foods that the Harvard School of Public Health cites as an example of a diet that is beneficial for warding off diabetes because of its high monounsaturated and polyunsaturated fat content.

Olive oil consumption was connected to a lower risk of developing diabetes in women, according to another study that was published in The American Journal of Clinical Nutrition.

Tip: Prevents Alzheimer's
The journal Scientific American claims that the oleocanthal found in olive oil can aid in the prevention of Alzheimer's disease. The American Chemical Society has also produced research with very comparable results.

In a study conducted in the United States, extra virgin olive oil was found to increase learning and memory in mice, lending credence to the hypothesis that this effect could be replicated in people who suffer from Alzheimer's disease.

Tip: Strengthens Bones

If you believed calcium was the only factor in bone health, think again. It may come as a surprise, but olive oil can also help strengthen the bones.
Olive oil was discovered to possibly contribute to men's bone health in a study that involved those individuals having a diet similar to that of the Mediterranean. It was discovered that their blood contained higher levels of osteocalcin, which was an indicator of good bone development.

Tip: Maintains Cholesterol Levels In Check

Is it true that olive oil lowers cholesterol levels? Olive oil use, on the other hand, is associated with a reduction in levels of "bad" cholesterol in the body. But does olive oil have a lot of cholesterol in it?

Olive oil has only trace amounts of both saturated and polyunsaturated lipids in its composition.

Because of this property, it has the power to manage the amounts of cholesterol in the blood that are found in the body. Olive oil has the largest concentration of monounsaturated fat, which ranges anywhere between 75 and 80 percent and contributes to the body's production of HDL and good cholesterol.

Oh no, I'm not going to assert this as a fact without any supporting scientific evidence.
Greek, Cretan, and other Mediterranean populations had much lower incidences of heart disease, according to research that was carried out at the University of Minnesota. This was the case even though these populations consumed virtually as much dietary fat as Americans do. The consumption of olive oil that is extra virgin in the Mediterranean region is being pointed out as the difference.
A study conducted at the Autonomous University of Madrid in Spain discovered that eating a diet high in extra virgin olive oil helped reduce the

levels of LDL cholesterol present in the body. It is also connected to a rise in HDL, generally known as the "good cholesterol," in the body of a person.

Tip: Helps Dilute Ear Wax

It's a smart move to clean ear wax with olive oil if you ask us.

Olive oil is often recommended as the method of choice for removing wax from ears by medical professionals to forestall the development of cerumen impaction. When you make an effort to clear impacted earwax, the chunks of hardened wax typically travel further into the ear canal as a result of your efforts.

Olive oil is extremely useful in situations like these. It will help to soften the cerumen, which will make it much simpler for you to remove the earwax. Once it has been sufficiently softened, the wax will begin to break down into smaller pieces. It will then typically go to the outer edge of your air canal, where it may be cleaned carefully and thoroughly using a soft cloth or tissue.

What Is Required Of You

Warm a tiny quantity of the oil to a temperature just slightly higher than room temperature. Earwax can be more easily removed with the use of warm olive oil. Be careful not to let it become too hot since this could cause your ear canal to burn. It shouldn't be any hotter than your body temperature, but it should be close to that.

Put a few drops of the oil into a clean dropper, and then turn it upside down. You won't need more than three-quarters of a dropper of a regular size.

Allow the oil to enter your ear canal slowly and gently. Make sure that your head is cocked to the side and that your ears are facing upwards by tilting your head. First, add just one drop, and if the consistency seems appropriate, continue to slowly add the rest of the oil.

Allow the oil to work for around ten to fifteen minutes before interfering. To improve the oil's ability to penetrate, change the position of your ear canal by softly opening and closing your mouth. You might also try massaging the region directly below your ear. If you feel the need to move about, placing a cotton swab over your ear can prevent the oil from leaking out of your ear.

When the earwax has been sufficiently loosened by the oil, turn your head so that the oil may drain out. You can clean it by using a dropper filled with warm water to flush the oil out, which will allow it to be rinsed away. While you are bathing, another option is to allow water to enter your ear canal and then wait for it to drain out.

At this point, you should use a gentle tissue or towel to remove any extra oil from the external portion of your ear.

You are free to carry out this procedure on a daily, weekly, or more frequent basis as needed. Some people believe that it should be done anywhere from two to four times each day, while others believe that the treatment should only be performed a few times per week. Because it may take up to two weeks for even mild cases to clear up after using this cure, you will need to exercise some patience.

Tip: Perks Up Sex Life

Have you ever wondered why all the great love stories began in Italy, the country that is famous for its olive oil?

Olive oil's reputation as a powerful aphrodisiac comes as no great surprise. When performed correctly, a massage with olive oil improves blood circulation to all regions of the body, including the genitourinary system.

CHAPTER 5

Tip: Alleviates The Symptoms Of Constipation:Olive Oil Can Be Utilized In A Variety Of Different Ways, Each Of Which Is Effective In Treating Constipation. Take A Look

Olive oil can be used as a treatment for those who suffer from constipation.

Olive oil is beneficial to the digestive system as well as the colon. Olive oil has a viscosity and texture that help stimulate your digestive system and make it easier for food to flow through the colon. When consumed consistently, this oil can fully eliminate the risk of developing constipation. The monounsaturated fat content of olive oil is particularly high. This helps to increase mobility, which is necessary for the colon to function properly and allow food to travel through it without obstruction. Additionally, it assists in the acceleration of bowel evacuation and protects against constipation.

This oil is an excellent source of a variety of nutrients, including vitamins E and K, iron, omega-3 and omega-6 fatty acids, and antioxidants. These nutrients not only boost your general health, which includes the health of your digestive tract, but they also aid in the prevention of constipation.

Olive Oil Can Be Utilized In A Variety Of Different Ways, Each Of Which Is Effective In Treating Constipation. Take A Look

1. Olive Oil Unrefined

Consume one tablespoon of extra virgin olive oil on two separate occasions per day. You should consume the first tablespoon on an empty stomach first thing in the morning, followed by the second one an hour before you go to bed. Wait a few hours after you have eaten before taking it, just in case you forget to take it when your stomach is empty. Do this daily until you no longer suffer from constipation.

2. Olive Oil Infused With Various Fruits

If you do not enjoy the flavor of raw olive oil, you can mask it by mixing it with a fruit that is high in fiber, such as an apple or an orange. After you have consumed the fruit, you should then take a spoonful of the oil first thing in the morning. If you find that it does not help, try taking an additional tablespoon of it in the evening along with some high-fiber vegetables like broccoli. Repeat this process consistently until you feel some alleviation.

3. Blended with Orange Juice and Olive Oil

Consume this mixture first thing in the morning on an empty stomach, adding one teaspoon of olive oil to one glass of orange juice. It will assist keep your system lubricated and will keep you healthy throughout the day. You might also try a tablespoon of olive oil mixed into your morning coffee.

4. Olive Oil Mixed With Fresh-Squeezed Lemon Juice

Another excellent natural treatment for constipation is to combine one tablespoon of olive oil with one teaspoon of lemon juice and mix the two. Consume this concoction once daily. You can also take one teaspoon of olive oil with a wedge of lemon in the evening to lubricate your system and prevent your colon from drying out as you sleep. Olive oil and lemon are both high in monounsaturated fats.

5. Blending Olive Oil and Milk

This is an excellent treatment for the most severe cases of constipation. All that is required of you is to combine one tablespoon of unrefined olive oil from extra virgin olive oil with one cup of warm milk. It should be thoroughly mixed, and before you consume it, you should make sure your stomach is empty. Constipation can be alleviated by doing this regularly.

CHAPTER

When Selecting Olive Oil, Five Key Considerations Should Be At The Forefront Of Your Mind.

#1. Checking to see if the olive oil is an extra virgin is the first thing you need to do before using it. Look for the phrase "extra virgin" on the back of the bottle after you have turned it around. However, there are several other factors to consider.

#2. Make sure you know where the oil came from. The oil has traveled a long way before reaching the store if you see a lot of countries stated on the backside label of the bottle. Additionally, there is a high potential that the oil has deteriorated as a result of this long journey.

#3. Check the date that it was harvested. It is essential to keep in mind that, unlike wine, olive oil does not improve with age. This is a key difference. If the oil is kept in ideal conditions, it has a potential shelf life of roughly two years (inside a dark cupboard at room temperature). If you can't find any indication of when the grapes were picked, you should probably put the bottle back where it came from and look into other options.

#4. Don't forget to take in the aroma and taste it. You won't be able to get away with that in the store. However, once you have brought the oil into your home, you should make it a point to both smell and taste a little bit of it. If the oil has an unpleasant smell, such as that of stale peanut butter, wax, or smelly socks, you should take it back to the retailer and tell them it has gone rancid.

#5. Favor domestic oil. Now, high-quality olive oil can be found in almost every region of the world. However, research has shown that olive oils produced in the nation of origin regularly score higher on quality scales than those imported from other countries.

Storage

It is just as crucial, if not more so, to properly store a product after it has been selected.

Take notice of these basic guidelines to ensure that your olive oil will last as long as possible.

When looking for a spot to store the oil, look for one that is cool and dark.

Make sure the oil is stored in a cool, dark place away from heat, air, and light.

The oil should be kept in a dark or opaque glass bottle, or a container made of stainless steel.

Check that the bottle's cap is securely fastened before using it.

The typical shelf life of cooking oils is shorter than that of olive oil, which is a blessing because olive oil may be stored for a longer period. There are even some that can survive for three years.

Using Olive Oil In The Kitchens

You can use extra virgin olive oil of the highest quality as a great condiment by drizzling it over fish, vegetables that have been steamed or baked, salad dressings, bread, cookies, and other foods.

It is vital to keep in mind that olive oil, in comparison to other oils, has a lower smoke point. The smoke point refers to the temperature at which the oil begins to degrade and lose its therapeutic properties. In addition, the smoke point of extra virgin olive oil is lower than that of regular olive oil. Make sure that when you are cooking on medium or low heat you are using extra virgin olive oil (between 250 to 350 degrees Fahrenheit).

A Strong Word Of Warning

Even though olive oil provides a lot of benefits, you can't overlook the fact that it also has some adverse effects because they're too important.

Take a look:

Certain people are more likely to have allergic reactions to olive oil than others. When olive oil is applied to the skin of a person who is allergic to olive oil, the immune system reacts by launching an attack on the oil. This results in the production of antibodies within the body, which creates symptoms that are typical of food allergies.

Those who are allergic to olive oil are at risk of developing eczema and other skin rashes, both of which have the potential to be irritating. Because of this, you should always do a patch test before applying the oil topically to your skin. If you experience any kind of allergic reaction, you should visit your allergist or dermatologist as soon as possible.

Because of the high caloric content of olive oil, consuming excessive amounts of it can increase the risk of heart disease. You must limit your daily consumption of olive oil to no more than two tablespoons.

Before using oil, you should discuss your condition with your physician if you have diabetes and are currently taking prescribed treatment. Olive oil may induce a reaction with the medications you are taking, leading to a further drop in your blood sugar levels. This can be quite dangerous.

Olive oil consumption that exceeds the recommended amount can result in several adverse health effects, including a precipitous drop in blood pressure, obstruction of the gallbladder, and various other disorders.

Because olive oil contains a high percentage of fat, consuming too much of it may have the opposite effect on your weight than what you were hoping for.

It is important not to heat olive oil for too long (more than 20 to 30 seconds) since the oil has a propensity to burn easily, which causes it to lose the majority of its health benefits.

Never apply the oil directly to cuts or wounds without first consulting a professional.

When cooking for pregnant or breastfeeding women, reduce the amount of oil used in the recipe.

CONCLUSION

Olive oil can be used to achieve skin that is perfect, smooth, and soft. Applying a small amount of this oil to your lips and heels will help make them more even and attractive. This one-of-a-kind oil not only makes your hair healthy but also makes it shine. Olive oil has also been shown to be particularly useful in the treatment of kidney stones, cholesterol, diabetes, breast cancer, cardiovascular disease, and obesity.

Olive oil is a ubiquitous component in both the culinary world and the world of personal care products. Iron, antioxidants, vitamins E and K, omega-3 fatty acids, and omega-6 fatty acids are all abundant in this oil. Olive oil use helps to moisturize the skin, maintains healthy hair and nails, lowers the risk of breast cancer and diabetes, and strengthens bones. Olive oil also reduces the risk of cardiovascular disease. On the other hand, certain people can have allergic reactions to it, and excessive consumption of it may raise the chance of developing heart disease. As a result, you should drink it in moderation and talk to your physician in the event of any unexpected complications.